Stop Malaria. Read This Book.

Olatundun Solomon

olatundunsolomon@gmail.com

Malaria is fever that
occur to the body.
The body
temperature is high
above normal body
temperature. Malaria
occur to the body
when female
anopheles mosquito
bites the body and

put plasmodium into the body. Plasmodium is parasite, it feeds from the blood and cause harm to the human body. Plasmodium parasites are: Plasmodium vivax, plasmodium falciparu m, Plasmodium ovale, and also Plasmodium malariae. The human body blood flows as the heart continue to beat. When the red blood cell is infected, if not treated it can lead to other red blood cells to be infected. When other red blood cells are infected, it can lead to anemia. To know if it is malaria, there should be laboratory test in the hospital. When animal is infected, mosquito can bite the animal and then bite human. Therefore, malaria can be transmitted from animal to human after the mosquito as bitten the animal and then bite human. Malaria can occur to somebody in the hospital by the use of already used syringes of somebody that is infected by malaria to another person that is not affected by malaria parasite. So therefore, it is expected to use new

syringes on patients
and not already used
syringes. Female
anopheles mosquito
that has malaria
parasites can bite
somebody wearing
short sleeves clothes
outside the house at
night. The mosquito

can bite the forearms and also the hands. It is therefore, advisable to wear long sleeve clothes outside the house and also wear hand gloves outside the house at night.

<u>Signs And Symptoms Of Malaria:</u>

Malaria fever can cause yellow skin and eyes when jaundice occur. It cause fever, that is the temperature of the body is above normal body temperature. It can cause vomiting. It can cause fatigue. It can also cause headache. It can cause weight loss. It can cause undernutrition.

Shivering can also occur to the body.

When these signs and symptoms begins to occur, it is very important to go to the hospital for diagnosis and treatment. The earlier the diagnosis and treatment, it can

make earlier

treatment to occur.

When not going to

the hospital early can

cause dangerous

happenings to occur

to the body. It can

lead to large

complications that

can lead to more and more time of treatment. Because the more the complications increases, it can lead to more organs and parts of the body to be infected. So therefore, it is necessary to start the

treatment very early.

<u>Prevention:</u>

Malaria can be prevented using mosquito nets. This net protect the body. It can be used to cover the windows. It can be used on the doors. It can be used to cover the bed.

Adding sliding glass windows to the house and glass doors can aid protection to prevent mosquito. Making sure that there is no stagnant water in the ground can prevent mosquito breeding areas. Using pesticides to spray around the house can prevent malaria. It is advisable to have proper environmental sanitation, by keeping the environment clean.

Inside the house fumigation method is also used. But when the house is fumigated, it is expected to go outside the house until the fumigation chemical subsides. This is because the

fumigation chemical
can be dangerous to
health.

<u>Treatment Of Malaria:</u>

Malaria is treated by the use of antimalarial drug.

Malaria can also be treated by the use of King of bitters leaf. King of bitters leaf can be chewed and swallowed. The taste is very bitter, but it is very effective.

Malaria can also be treated by drinking the chlorophyll of Vernonia amygdalina. It is known as bitter leaf. The chlorophyll is gotten by washing the leaves with water,

then carrying the
leaves into a dry bowl
and squeeze it
continuously. It will
then cause green
liquid to drop into the
bowl. Drinking the
chlorophyll of
Vernonia amygdalina

can be used to treat malaria.

Also taking lime juice and honey mixed together and drink it can be used to treat malaria.